Published By Adam Gilbin

@ Terry Plant

Change Your Habits: Transform Your Life

With New Habits

All Right RESERVED

ISBN 978-87-94477-59-8

TABLE OF CONTENTS

chapter 1 1

What Are Human Habits?... 1

Chapter 2 6

Little Propensities For Improved Efficiency And Work 6

Chapter 3 11

Looking At Existing Habits 11

Chapter 4 16

How To Break Bad Habits 16

Chapter 5 24

Develop A Consistent Wake-Up Routine....................... 24

What Are Habits And How Are They Formed?.............. 36

Chapter 6 40

The Power Of Habits 40

Chapter 7 44

The Science Of Habits: Unveiling The Foundation 44

Chapter 8 48

Spiral – How Habits Work 48

Chapter 9	54
Understanding The Habit Loop	54
Chapter 10	64
How Small Changes Can Trigger Big Transformation	64
Chapter 11	72
Introduction To Behavioral Transformation	72
Understanding The Foundations Of Behavioral Health	72
Chapter 12	85
Your Spiritual Challenge	85
Chapter 13	88
Potentially Good Habits To Add Spirituality To Your Life	88
Chapter 14	92
How Can Habits Change My Life?	92
Chapter 15	100
Challenge Yourself	100
Chapter 16	107
Creating Productive Habits	107

Choose Habits That Align With Your Goals 107

Chapter 17 119

Identifying Bad Habits 119

Recognizing Barriers To Change 119

Chapter 18 130

The Power Of Rituals And Keystone Habits 130

Keystone Habits: Unleashing Domino Effects 133

Chapter 19 137

Neurology, Willpower And Habit Change 137

Chapter 9	Understanding The Habit Loop	54
Chapter 10	How Small Changes Can Trigger Big Transformation	64
Chapter 11	Introduction To Behavioral Transformation	72
	Understanding The Foundations Of Behavioral Health	72
Chapter 12	Your Spiritual Challenge	85
Chapter 13	Potentially Good Habits To Add Spirituality To Your Life	88
Chapter 14	How Can Habits Change My Life?	92
Chapter 15	Challenge Yourself	100
Chapter 16	Creating Productive Habits	107

Choose Habits That Align With Your Goals 107

Chapter 17 119

Identifying Bad Habits 119

Recognizing Barriers To Change 119

Chapter 18 130

The Power Of Rituals And Keystone Habits 130

Keystone Habits: Unleashing Domino Effects 133

Chapter 19 137

Neurology, Willpower And Habit Change 137

CHAPTER 1

What are human habits?

Habit is an action that is performed by itself, without the participation of our will. These are patterns of behavior that have developed over time. We are not born with ready habits. Habits are the result of our own, once made choice, repeatedly repeated and brought to automatism. First, we create our own habits, and then our habits create our life.

In the modern world there are a huge number of moments that require our attention, the attention of our consciousness, our operational memory. It may be other people, information, own thoughts, and so on. Therefore, it would be waste of our time to pay attention to thinking about the little things, for example, about the sequence of cleaning teeth: first, the upper left, then the lower left, then the front one etc... Plus, conscious cleansing would take more time than unconscious. Our habits of doing the necessary daily routines, as in the example above, without thinking about them, release our memory and our time for making more important decisions. Therefore, the habits are more important for us than ever before in our busy life.

Habit is an inner need as a reaction to circumstances. For example, before going to bed, you go brushing your teeth. The circumstances in this case are the evening and the house (time and place) and the need - to brush your teeth. If brushing your teeth is not a habit, then you need an effort to remember to brush your teeth, decide whether to do it or not, and force yourself to do so. When an action has already become a habit, it is easy for you to perform it. We do our usual actions without thinking about them.

For forming a new habit you need motivation. Motivation is not a constant thing. When you want to start doing something useful, it often happens that today you have the motivation to perform this action that in the future will lead you to some positive changes, but it takes just a couple of days, maybe a week, and your motivation ends.

And if by the time, when your motivation is over, you have developed a habit - then this action (habit) will continue to be performed. Sometimes, when there is not enough motivation, you, of course, can force yourselves to do something through willpower. But unfortunately, willpower is also often not enough.

Will-power is the ultimate resource, which means that will-power has the property of ending. And if the action has not become a habit, then it takes a huge amount of this resource, and sometimes it turns out that at the moment you don't have enough of it.

Unfortunately, the usual habits that we are trying to create simply by repetition do not have time to develop in 5-7 days; it takes much more time to develop them.

In this book you will get acquainted with a system that will allow you to reduce the period of habit development to a minimum, literally up to a week. Moreover, already in 3 - 5 days you will see that the habit has practically been formed and does not require almost any effort from you.

Habits quietly and effortlessly improve our quality of life. Habits quietly and effortlessly improve our quality of life. The beauty of habits is that we, once having formed them, after a certain number of months or years, notice that there have been some positive changes in our life. And at the same time they occurred unnoticed, practically no effort was required of us, to be more precisely - the efforts were required only at the stage of formation of habits.

CHAPTER 2

Little Propensities for Improved Efficiency and Work

Do a 5-minute day to day survey at your work area by the day's end.

Before you go home, or from your work area, at home before you wrap things up for the afternoon (or night!), *require five minutes*.

Record what you achieved in a fast, bulleted list. Record what you didn't achieve that you had expected to, and what halted you. Try not to pummel yourself for your disappointments, simply notice, in the event that you can, what made you become derailed.

Furthermore, notice the amount of work or progress you achieved. This sort of survey is a method for assisting your mind with zeroing in on the positive (I achieved something today) and will assist you with turning out to be more mindful of the things that will more often than not wreck you or divert you from useful work.

Claim to be your legend.

Whenever you're confronted with a difficult circumstance, a scary venture, another professional jump, a significant gathering, ponder a legend in your industry or vocation. Then ask yourself what this individual would do in your circumstance.

How might she deal with it? Could he be scared? Unfortunate? Or then again certain and quiet? Presently envision yourself doing the exact thing you think your legend would do. This assists with explaining that the smart activities are for you by eliminating one's uncertainty and negative self-talk that can impede you in vulnerability.

Switch off all notices, for somewhere around one long square of work-time, consistently.

Our cerebrums are not proficient at changing; starting with one undertaking then onto the next.

The single ding of an email warning or text, regardless of whether it's tied in with something totally immaterial, can make you lose up to 40% of your work time. Is it truly worth the effort?

Let's just imagine that you have endless time available to you. Yet we realize that you don't. Do yourself as well and your profession some help, and quieten every one of the dings and tweets for something like one long square of time .

Go through 5 minutes daily contemplating the cycle you will take that will get you to your professional objectives.

This is the right sort of certain perception. Imagining the final product doesn't normally assist you with arriving. Yet, imagining yourself doing the means you will take to arrive at your ultimate objective can assist you with really finishing those means when the time has come.

Answer all solicitations and open doors with "I'll really look at my schedule."

Stop the automatic reaction that you give, whether it is negative or positive.

Perhaps you're excessively fast to say no. Or then again perhaps you're an accommodating person and you're excessively speedy to say OK, and regard yourself as over-booked and overpowered.

Offer yourself an opportunity to assess each chance by essentially making it your training not to answer immediately. All things being equal, say, "I'll check my schedule and let you know."

Then, when you make some little memories, really take a look at your schedule, your needs, and figure out what you can fit it in.

Chapter 3

Looking at Existing Habits

In this chapter, we take a look at the normal seemingly boring things that you do every day of your life. You will need to take pen and paper and give yourself about half an hour to sit down and write out all the things that are the monotonous routines that you do without thinking. In fact, if you would rather, why not carry a notepad with you for an entire day and simply note down the habits that you incorporate into your everyday life. You may be asking yourself what kind of habits, but let's explain.

When you get out of bed in the morning, what do you normally do? You may instinctively reach for your slippers. You may go to the lavatory. You may go to the bathroom and clean your teeth. These are all habits. You may then wander into the kitchen and make a coffee. You may go to open your letters. You will most certainly get dressed.

These are habits and these can all be used to piggyback new habits. You need to be able to make a list of these so that they can be used in the piggyback process, but don't write down the things you SHOULD do. Write down the things you DO. There is a difference because with all of the good intentions in the world, if the item you have chosen is not already a habit, you will fail. You need real habits and positive ones so that you can use these as triggers for incorporating new habits. For example, you may think that exercise should be part of your morning routine, but may have failed to exercise because you found other things to do. If you have intentions rather than habits, don't include these because they are not habits at this moment in time.

The next thing that you need to do is make a list of habits that would improve your life. You know what they are because you live your life. Perhaps you don't make enough time to keep in touch with people or perhaps you smoke too much. Perhaps you don't drink as much water as you should. Perhaps you tend to get distracted easily and want to concentrate more. Write down your list and try to include the following:

- Be friendlier
- Be healthier
- Be more empathetic
- Socialize more
- Have a spiritual moment
- Relax more

I have written out these so that you can see from the knowledge you have of your own life which areas of your life you need to improve. That's important and it's also important that you are honest with yourself. Perhaps you are not good with people and wish that you were. In that case, add the habit of socializing more. Perhaps you don't see the spiritual side of life and if that's the case, add the spirituality habit. Perhaps you are tense and always stressed. In that case, add the relaxation habit. Perhaps you are standoffish and see yourself as unpopular. Add the "Be friendlier" habit. We can break these areas of habits into smaller and more manageable habits later, but you need to admit where your life is not giving you sufficient satisfaction, as each of these areas will encompass habits that can be piggybacked onto existing habits to make your life more complete. Now, we can look at specific areas and show you how to incorporate 30 new habits into your life over the period of 30 days and make them stick. It's up to you how many you introduce at a time, but keep a note of them and begin to tick them off every day that you perform these new habits. By tagging them onto old and established habits, you are giving yourself a prompt that will help you to understand exactly when to introduce that new habit.

CHAPTER 4

HOW TO BREAK BAD HABITS

Breaking bad habits can be easy when you go into the task armed with the right information. There are tons of different ways you can work on improving your bad habits and replacing them with good ones instead. Some methods might work better for you than others, so don't be afraid to try a little bit of everything to see what keeps you on the right path to success. In no time, you'll start seeing some impressive changes in your life, all thanks to your attention to your bad habits.

Set realistic goals

First and foremost, set realistic goals for yourself. Every bad habit has to be broken down into stages, and it's important to work in small steps before you try to jump into the bigger picture.

Remember that bad habits have cues, behaviors, and rewards, and try to break each one of your habits into these categories to figure out where to get started.

Rebecca is a nail-biter. She's been biting her nails since she was in the first grade, and now that she's in her thirties, she's ready to have healthy fingernails for once in her life. Unfortunately, this bad habit is so ingrained in her psyche that she doesn't know how to get started.

Rebecca can tell that the cue that causes her to bite her nails is her nervousness, and the reward is the sense that she's in control of something when she chews on her fingernails. Her first goal should be to find some other way of feeling in control, like holding a worry stone instead. After that, she can break her habit down into smaller steps, and slowly work toward growing her fingernails out long and healthy again.

Stay focused

Keep focused on your goals every step of the way to fight off your bad habits successfully. If you lose focus, you'll be back at square one in no time, and you'll have to start all over again.

Rebecca, for example, would have to start growing her fingernails from the ground up if she lost focus and started biting them again. If this happens, don't let yourself get discouraged. Just dust yourself off, get up, and try again.

Work with a friend or family member

Having a "bad habit buddy" can work wonders for keeping you accountable on your journey to breaking these behaviors. If you have a trusted friend or family member, ask them if they'll be your partner and maybe even try to break a few of their bad habits, too. When you work with someone, it's much easier to be happy about your accomplished goals, and to question yourself before sliding into a setback.

Rebecca's sister Maria is trying to stop spending too much money on clothes, shoes, and other unnecessary items every month. The two of them work together to break their bad habits by offering support when needed and sharing in each other's triumphs. They talk twice a week about how things are going, and it's a huge help to both of them.

Keep a record

Write down how things go every time you work on breaking your bad habit. It's a good idea to keep a chart listing out each day of the week and specifying your strengths, weaknesses, and new goals. This way, if you ever feel discouraged, you can look back over your notes and see how far you've come.

As Rebecca has worked on her nail-biting habit, she's kept notes on her goals and achievements. She also writes down every time something makes her nervous enough to want to bite her nails again. When she finally grew them out long enough to paint them for the first time in years, she wrote that down, too. Now she can look back on her progress and notice patterns of ups and downs.

Forgive yourself for mistakes

Everybody makes mistakes! It's okay if you make mistakes along the way. Some bad habits are a lot easier to break than others, and if you struggle for a long time with your worst ones, there's no shame in that. Smoking is a bad habit that can sometimes take years to stop, and even then, it's always tempting to backslide. If you find yourself making mistakes frequently, you might want to change tracks and come at your bad habits from a different angle. Mistakes every now and then, however, are nothing more than chances to learn about what works and what doesn't.

Rebecca's first mistake in trying to quit biting her nails made her want to give up for good. She had been doing well, and had gone almost a whole week without biting. Then one night, she couldn't reach her sister on the phone at their usual time. She got worried about her sister and started biting her nails again. Only after her sister called her and said everything was fine did Rebecca realize she'd been biting. This setback was tough, since it made Rebecca feel like her progress had been for nothing. She reminded herself, however, that mistakes happen, and she kept pushing forward once again.

Try meditation

Meditation is a great way to work on breaking bad habits. When you meditate, you strengthen your mind and your willpower, and give yourself the ability to take control over your thoughts and actions. Even the worst of bad habits can be overcome with simple meditation techniques.

If you've never meditated before, don't worry! It's not too hard, especially with practice. Try an easy breathing meditation to get yourself in the right frame of mind. Follow these steps and you'll be meditating like a pro in no time:

Sit down with your back straight and your eyesclosed in a quiet place with no distractions.

There's no need to slow down your breathing for this exercise.

Count your breaths as your chest moves up and down.

Set a timer for 5 to 10 minutes to begin with.

Keeping your eyes closed, breathe at your normal rate.

Count one in, one out; two in, two out, and so on.

As you count, try to think of nothing but your breaths. If other thoughts come into your mind, push them away and keep your thoughts clear and free.

If you lose your place counting because you get distracted, start over.

It's okay if you can't concentrate all the way to ten breaths the first time you practice. It takes time to keep your mind clear. The more you work on this, the easier it will become to focus your thoughts and control your mind.

CHAPTER 5

DEVELOP A CONSISTENT WAKE-UP ROUTINE

Did you ever realize how powerful mornings are? There's a reason some of the most successful people in the world have committed morning routines that they wouldn't dare to skip.

It doesn't have to be getting up at 5am to make a protein-filled smoothie and going for an hour-long jog. It just means deciding how to best wake your body, mind, and soul up to begin your day.

The routine could be as small as committing to never hitting the snooze button again. It could incorporate a cup of warm lemon water, or simply writing down your goals for the day.

Whatever you decide, the key is to keep it consistent. Make your morning routine something you can make into a solid habit that you won't leave on the shelf.

If you're not a natural morning person, the first hours of the day can be rough. You're probably grumpy and tired, and just don't feel ready to deal with what the day has to offer. But if you want to make the most out of your entire day, it's important that you use your mornings wisely. If you can wake up early, feeling energized and ready to go, you'll set yourself up for a productive and successful day.

The first step to making your time dynamic and effective is to lay the groundwork with a routine that helps you create a rewarding and constructive morning. It all starts the moment you open your eyes. Use these 22 tips to ensure you wake up early, feeling energized and empowered.

1. Have an intentional nighttime routine.

Waking up feeling refreshed and energized begins with your habits the night before. Build an intentional nighttime routine that helps you relax and sets you up for sleep. Take a few minutes to prepare for the next day, such as laying out clothes to wear for the upcoming day or having your workout gear ready to go if you plan to go to the gym.

2. Take a minute to tidy up before bed.

Nothing is quite as demotivating as waking up to a sink full of dirty dishes or a messy room with clothes scattered everywhere. Take a few minutes before bed to organize and tidy up your living spaces. You'll wake up feeling more refreshed because everything is neat and orderly. This will help you feel like each day is a fresh start and a chance to begin anew.

3. Make your bedtime thoughts positive ones.

Before you go to sleep, tell yourself that you're going to wake up feeling refreshed and that you're looking forward to tomorrow. Go to bed with positive thoughts about the next day. You program yourself to wake up feeling happy and energized. This may seem like a small thing, but your first thoughts in the morning often reflect the last thoughts you had before falling asleep. It can change your entire day.

4. Sleep rituals.

Bedtime rituals are habits that signal to your brain that it's time for bed. These should be small, calming activities that quiet your mind and allow you to wind down. They might include making a cup of chamomile tea, reading a book before sleep, or a simple ten minute meditation.

5. Unplug and decompress.

If you want to feel amazing in the morning, it's important to allow yourself to decompress and unplug before bed. Stop checking e-mails and avoid social media for at least an hour before sleep. Instead, spend some time reflecting on your day and thinking about what possibilities are you excited for tomorrow.

6. Develop a consistent sleep schedule.

By consistently going to bed and getting up at about the same time every day, your body will know what to expect -- when it's time for sleep and when it's time to rise. You should aim to get your ideal amount of sleep most nights -- usually somewhere between seven and nine hours.

7. Have a positive morning ritual.

Many successful people and high achievers are early birds who get a ton done before most people have even taken their first sip of coffee. But, as Hal Elrod describes in What positive morning ritual would help elevate your desires in your mind and your body to act upon those desires?

8. Don't hit the snooze button.

Many of us are guilty of hitting the snooze button when the alarm blares us awake. Our beds feel so cozy, and it's easy to want to doze off for a few more minutes. However, hitting snooze signals that you're not ready for your day. You're robbing yourself of valuable time that can be used for your sense of purpose.

9. Wake up determined each day.

If you get up every day with a sense of ambition and feeling determined to make something of your day, you're setting yourself up for a satisfying day. Start your day with intention and feel motivated to jump right into it.

10. Treat every morning like Christmas.

If you constantly feel sluggish and humdrum in the morning, try changing the way you approach your day by changing your attitude about sleep. For instance, were you ever tired on Christmas morning as a kid, even if you didn't get a lot of sleep? Of course not! That's because you woke up excited. Even though you didn't get enough sleep, you weren't about to slow down. It's the creation of new, positive habits.

11. Try placebo sleep.

It's hard to get energized if you wake up feeling cranky. You do this to yourself when you constantly tell yourself you're exhausted. Try some placebo sleep for a quick pick-me-up. Tell yourself you feel well rested and that you're energized and ready to go. Your mind will program your body to follow suit. The body is not in control. It is your mind where it all begins.

12. Move your alarm clock across the room.

By moving your alarm clock across the room, you'll force yourself to get up to turn it off. This will reduce the urge to go back to sleep, as it will get you up and moving first thing in the morning.

13. Start small.

Keep your morning routine short and easy to accomplish. If you have a huge checklist of things you have to do every morning, it's no wonder you feel overwhelmed and exhausted before you even get out of bed. If you keep your morning routine simple, you'll be more apt to stick to it. It will start your day feeling relaxed, composed, and ready for all possibilities.

14. Stack your habits.

Make sure you build your morning routine in such a way that you're consistently creating a positive day for yourself. Your routine should not only be about getting ready. It should be about building you up for your day full of possibilities.

15. Create peace and calm in your morning.

Don't allow stress and anxiety to wreak havoc to your morning. Quiet your mind by making time for purposeful silence. This is a chance to engage in meditation, practice mindfulness, or even just sit quietly and allow yourself to feel peaceful. Start with five minutes and increase the length over time. You will begin to realize how important it is to start within to execute all you desire in the 3-D world.

16. Reflect and feel gratitude.

As part of this practice of finding peace in your morning, take a moment to reflect on your life and all the things you're grateful for. Starting your day with gratitude can change your entire perspective and influence how you react and make decisions.

17. Banish your cell phone from your bedside.

Take a tip from Arianna Huffington: "When it's time for sleep, put your cell phone away at night." Huffington keeps it out of her bedroom altogether or put it in airplane mode.

18. Keep your mornings light on electronics.

Another benefit to keeping your phone out of your room is that you won't be tempted to check e-mail or social media first thing in the morning. Doing this helps keep stress and anxiety from invading your morning. Don't distract yourself by starting your day responding to other people's needs. Start your day on your terms.

19. Do what is meaningful to you.

Do what is meaningful to you in the morning, and you'll set a positive tone for your whole day. If that means going for a run because you value exercise and want to get it done, then do that. If you value spending time with your family, then make time for your family. You are the creator of your own reality.

20. No morning is a failure.

For some mornings, you won't be able to stick to your routine. Something will come up, something will throw you off, and you won't be able to do things the way you normally would. That's okay. Be flexible, and recognize that disruption in your morning routine is inevitable -- it doesn't mean your whole day is ruined.

21. Make your mornings pro-active.

Start your day with a pro-active mindset. Make your mornings about your own needs and goals, and schedule your day, accordingly. Begin by knocking off at least one task that's on your high-priority list.

22. See what really works for you.

The key to crafting the perfect morning regimen is to experiment with what works best for you. Try out different routines and see what makes you happy. Some things will work better for certain people than for others -- be open to shaping your morning around what works for you. The morning is the fuel to your day. Make sure you go through trial and error for what works best for your mind, body, and soul.

What are habits and how are they formed?
Habits are patterns of behavior that are acquired through repetition. They are the actions we perform almost automatically, without conscious or deliberate effort. This ability to act without prior deliberation is what makes habits so powerful in our lives. Their influence is so profound that habits often dictate the way we live, work and play, shaping our lives in ways we barely notice.

The formation of a habit begins with a conscious decision. In the beginning, an action requires deliberate effort and active decision making. For example, if you decide to start exercising, the first few days or weeks may require significant conscious effort. However, over time, this action becomes a more natural and fluid part of your daily routine. Exercise no longer requires the same amount of conscious effort or deliberation. This transition from conscious effort to automation is at the heart of the habit-forming process.

The human brain, always in search of efficiency, converts these repeated actions into habits to conserve mental energy. In doing so, it frees up cognitive resources for other tasks that require greater attention and deliberation. This efficiency is a double sword, as it can also lead to the formation of unwanted or negative habits just as easily as positive habits.

Habit formation can best be understood through the concept of "habit loops," which are composed of three elements: trigger, routine, and reward. The trigger is the event or circumstance that initiates the habit. For example, the sound of an alarm in the morning may be the trigger for a morning exercise routine. The routine is the action or behavior itself, such as running or yoga.

The reward is the benefit you get from performing the routine, such as feeling more energized or having a better mood.

Over time, this trigger-routine-reward cycle becomes stronger. The brain begins to anticipate the reward even before the routine is completed, which increases the likelihood that the routine will be executed when the trigger is presented. This process is what ultimately makes habits so powerful and, at times, difficult to change.

It is important to note that habits are not only formed in the realm of physical actions. They are also formed in our way of thinking and in our emotional responses. For example, the tendency to worry in stressful situations can become a mental habit. Similarly, the way we respond emotionally to certain triggers, such as anger or frustration, can also be the result of emotional habits.

Understanding how habits are formed is critical to being able to modify them. By recognizing the components of the habit loop - trigger, routine, reward - we can begin to dismantle unwanted habits and build new habits that are more aligned with our goals and aspirations. This knowledge is especially relevant when we seek to improve our productivity and well-being, as habits play a central role in how we structure our time and daily actions.

In short, habits are more than just actions; they are the pillars on which we build our daily lives. Through understanding and conscious manipulation of habits, we can exercise greater control over our lives, increase our efficiency and improve our overall well-being. Habit formation is a powerful process, and with the right guidance and tools, we can shape our habits to better reflect our personal goals and values.

Chapter 6

The Power of Habits

Discovering the Secret to a Better Life

Habits are like the backbone of our lives. They shape our daily routine, influence our choices, and ultimately determine our success and happiness. However, many of us don't stop to consider how significant habits are in our lives. In this chapter, we'll explore in-depth what habits are, how they work, and why they're so crucial to achieving our goals and living the life of our dreams.

What are Habits?

Habits are automatic behaviors that we perform repeatedly without thinking much about them. They can be as simple as brushing your teeth every morning or as complex as following a regular exercise routine. The secret to habits is automation - they become a natural part of our daily lives.

The Habit Cycle

To better understand how habits work, it is essential to know the habit cycle. This cycle consists of three key elements:

1. Trigger: This is the first step in the cycle. A trigger is something that sets off the habit. It could be a specific time of day, an emotion, a place, or anything that triggers your brain to initiate automatic behavior.

2. Routine: Routine is the habitual action or behavior itself. It's what you do in response to the trigger. For example, if you feel stressed (trigger), you may resort to eating a snack (routine).

3. Reward: The reward is the gratification you receive after completing the routine. It satisfies a specific need or desire. In the previous example,

the reward might be a temporary feeling of relief from stress.

Why are Habits Important ?

Habits are powerful because, when developed well, they can lead to significant results. Here are some reasons why habits are crucial:

- Efficiency: Habits automate tasks, saving time and mental energy.

- Consistency: Habits help to maintain a desired behavior constantly.

- Gradual Progress: Small changes in habits can lead to big results over time.

- Continuous Improvement: Habits allow you to constantly evolve and grow.

- Achievement of Objectives: They are the key to achieving personal goals and objectives.

The Journey That Awaits Us

In this book, we'll explore how you can consciously shape your habits to improve your life. You'll learn how to identify and modify bad habits, set effective goals, and use behavioral science to your benefit. Along this journey, we'll share inspiring stories of real people who transformed their lives by forming good habits.

We're about to dive deep into the world of habits and discover how small changes can lead to big results. Get ready for a journey of self-discovery and personal growth. Our destiny? The success and fulfillment you deserve.

Before continuing, I kindly ask that after you complete this reading, you consider reviewing this book on Amazon . Your opinion is invaluable and can help other readers discover and benefit from this personal transformation guide. Let's continue our journey through the power of habits.

Chapter 7

The Science of Habits: Unveiling the Foundation

In this chapter, we will explore the science behind habits and uncover their fundamental aspects. By understanding the habit loop and how habits form, we can set the stage for building atomic habits that lead to lasting personal transformation.

The Habit Loop: Cue, Routine, Reward

Habits operate in a loop consisting of three key components: cue, routine, and reward. The cue is a trigger that signals our brain to initiate a specific habit. It can be a time of day, a location, an emotion, or even the presence of other people. The routine refers to the behavior itself, the actions we take in response to the cue. Lastly, the reward is the positive reinforcement we experience after completing the routine.

By recognizing the elements of the habit loop, we can gain insights into how habits are formed. Understanding this loop allows us to identify the cues that trigger our habits and the rewards that reinforce them.

The Brain's Role in Habit Formation

Our brain plays a crucial role in habit formation. Through a process called neuroplasticity, our brain builds connections that become stronger with repetitive actions. This enables habits to become ingrained in our daily lives. As we repeat a behavior, our brain begins to automate it, making it more efficient and less conscious.

Understanding the brain's role in habit formation empowers us to intentionally shape our behavior. By rewiring the neuronal connections in our brain, we can replace unwanted habits with new, positive ones.

Habit Stacking: Building upon Existing Habits

Habit stacking is a powerful technique that involves building new habits upon already established habits. By linking a new habit with an existing one, we leverage the power of automation and make it easier to adopt and maintain positive behaviors.

To implement habit stacking, we identify an existing habit that naturally occurs in our routine and use it as a cue to initiate a new habit. By connecting the two habits, we create a seamless integration that increases the likelihood of successfully implementing the new habit.

By understanding the habit loop, the brain's role in habit formation, and the strategy of habit stacking, we lay a strong foundation for building atomic habits. The following chapters will delve deeper into the specific laws and techniques that will guide us on our journey towards lasting personal transformation. So, let's proceed with enthusiasm and embrace the power of atomic habits!

Chapter 8

Spiral – How Habits Work

You wake up in a bad mood because it's late. You go to the bathroom and curse the bloated face and body you see in the mirror. You don't want to go to work because none of your clothes fit you, except for that shabby dress you wear at least three times a week. You don't like to shop for clothes because the clothes you like are not available in your size. You arrive in the office in a worse mood because you hadn't had time for breakfast and you're hungry. You're scared that your boss will yell at you again because the report due last week is still not finished. You don't feel like going out to lunch with your officemates because you don't like how you look compared to their chic office attires.

You just go somewhere else where you can smoke and eat a sandwich in peace. You go home tired and depressed. You go straight to the refrigerator to get the chocolate cake and ice cream – your comfort food. You stay in front of the TV way past midnight because you don't want to think about your miseries. The following morning, you wake up in a bad mood again because it's late.

Maybe you can relate with this story. Maybe you bought this eBook because you think you need to change some of your habits that stand between you and the kind of life you want to live. Perhaps you suddenly woke up one day and realized how far downhill your life has gone.

If we try to dissect the story above, we will be able to list down a number of things the girl in the story needs to do to change or eliminate her bad habits:

- **Wake up early**

- Work out to lose weight
- Avoid fattening foods
- Manage stress
- Quit staying up late watching TV
- Eat breakfast
- Manage time at work
- Quit smoking

This list can still get longer if we see more into the girl's life. But more than the length of the list, what needs to be noted is how one bad habit is linked to the next. The first bad habit of waking up late in the morning builds into two other bad habits of skipping breakfast and arriving late at work.

You may have experienced in your own life how just one bad habit can get you off track. Once you're off track, new bad habits sprout in your life one after the other. Before you know it, you've been sucked into a downward spiral and you suddenly find yourself with self-doubt, anxiety and stress.

The good news is that spirals go both ways – it can send you spiraling down or it can shoot spiraling up. If one bad habit can send you spiraling down, working on just one good habit can also shoot you spiraling up. Just one good habit is all it takes. Imagine how the story above will change if the girl woke up early for work instead.

She gets out of bed early. She feels good about herself. She goes to the bathroom and smiles at herself in the mirror. She tries on several outfits and finds out that she has enough clothes to mix and match for a polished look. She eats breakfast while planning her day at work. She gets to the office early and goes straight to her boss' room to discuss how she plans to meet her deliverables.

She goes out to lunch with her officemates and one of them tells her he could help in her report. She goes home with a feeling of accomplishment. She is in good spirits. She goes to the kitchen to prepare a decent dinner for herself. Later, she decides to go to bed early so she can have another good start tomorrow.

Yes, just one good habit can send you spiraling up. If you think you are in a desperate place right now, you can kick start your new life with just one habit change. This concept may be counter-intuitive if you have a long list of bad habits to break. But this is the most effective strategy because it will set you in motion.

- Starting with just one habit makes your life makeover manageable. You would agree that changing one habit is more achievable compared to changing 5 or 10 habits all at once.

- Having only one habit to change will give you full focus. You can pour all your energies into just one goal.

- Learning how to change one habit will inspire you and guide you in your next habit change.

Action Plan: Make your own list of bad habits to break or new habits to make. Choose one, an easy one. Then decide that you will give your 100% in changing that habit.

CHAPTER 9

UNDERSTANDING THE HABIT LOOP

Our everyday routines and conduct are both influenced by and shaped by our habits. Habits play a crucial role in our existence, whether it be the reflexive morning ritual of brewing coffee, the subliminal chewing of our fingernails during stressful situations, or the regular exercise regimen that keeps us fit. But what precisely is a habit, and how do these deeply established habits arise? The interesting realm of habits is thoroughly explored in this investigation, which also looks at how habits are defined, and formed, and how psychological processes contribute to them.

Habits are like the hidden gears that drive our daily lives. To comprehend their inner workings, we must first dissect the habit loop—a fundamental concept in habit formation. The habit loop consists of three key components: the cue, the routine, and the reward.

A recurrent behavior that is carried out automatically in response to a particular cue or trigger and requires little conscious thinking or effort can be widely referred to as a habit. These actions can be both beneficial, like frequent exercise, and harmful, such

The Cue: Every habit starts with a cue, also known as a trigger or a prompt. This is the signal that initiates the habit. Cues can be external, like the smell of freshly brewed coffee in the morning, or internal, such as feeling stressed or anxious. Identifying the cues that prompt your habits is crucial because it allows you to become more aware of your behavior.

External cues: These cues come from our immediate surroundings. They could be specific places or sensory inputs like sights, sounds, or smells. The smell of freshly baked cookies (which encourages munching) or the sound of your alarm clock (which prompts your morning ritual) are two examples of external cues.

Internal Cues: On the other hand, internal cues are caused by our mental or physiological conditions. They could include emotions like fear, boredom, or hunger. Our brains may unconsciously start habit-triggering behaviors as a coping mechanism or pleasurable behavior when we perceive these internal cues. For instance, stress may cause you to start chewing your nails, whereas hunger prompts you to eat.

Since cues are the starting point for habit formation, understanding them is essential. The craving that propels the habit loop onward is produced when the brain registers a cue and expects the related reward. Here are some essential tips about cues:

Recognition of Patterns: Humans are very adept at seeing trends and connecting signs to certain actions. For instance, over time, your brain comes to correlate the enjoyable experience of exercising with seeing your running shoes (an external cue). You are more inclined to follow your training regimen when you see such shoes because of this relationship.

Stacking Habits: Cues can be cleverly employed to create brand-new routines. Habit stacking, which involves connecting a new habit you want to form with an existing habit, is a well-liked habit-building technique. For instance, you can cue the new habit by placing your meditation cushion next to your toothbrush (an existing habit cue) if you wish to start practicing daily meditation but find it difficult to recall.

Consistency Matters: The more frequently a trigger is linked to a particular habit, the more solid the connection in your brain grows. Consistency feeds back into the habit loop, further automating the behavior.

Control and Awareness: The first stage in habit change is to become aware of your cues. You can take proactive measures to change bad habits or substitute healthier cues by identifying the factors that set them off.

In conclusion, cues are what trigger the development of habits. They can take many different shapes and influence our behaviors in both internal and external ways. Understanding the impact of cues enables us to not only identify and change old behaviors but also consciously form new ones that promote our well-being and personal development.

The Routine:

The routine is the habitual behavior itself—the action you take in response to the cue. It could be something as simple as reaching for your coffee mug or scrolling through your phone when you're stressed. This is the part of the habit that you're looking to change or modify.

The Reward:

The reward is what makes the habit loop complete. It's the positive outcome or feeling you gain from the routine. Your brain associates this reward with the cue and the routine, reinforcing the habit. For example, the caffeine in your morning coffee provides a sense of alertness and satisfaction, which reinforces the habit of drinking coffee.

Understanding the habit loop is like having a roadmap to your own behavior. By identifying the cues and rewards associated with your habits, you can begin to intervene and make deliberate changes to the routines. Whether you want to break a bad habit or establish a new one, manipulating the habit loop is a powerful tool in habit formation.

The Brain's Role in Habit Formation

Our brains are incredible learning machines and habit formation is no exception. The basal ganglia, a region deep within the brain, plays a pivotal role in this process. Here's how it works:

Cue Recognition:

When you encounter a cue, whether it's the aroma of your favorite meal or the ping of a notification on your phone, your brain's basal ganglia takes notice. It recognizes this cue as a trigger for a specific habit.

Habit Formation:

Once the cue is recognized, the basal ganglia sends a signal to the prefrontal cortex, another part of the brain responsible for decision-making and behavior. Initially, when you're forming a habit, the prefrontal cortex plays a significant role in decision-making. However, as the habit becomes ingrained, the prefrontal cortex's involvement decreases, and the habit becomes more automatic.

Reward sensation:

As you perform the habit's routine, your brain releases neurotransmitters, such as dopamine, which create a sense of pleasure or satisfaction. This positive reinforcement strengthens the habit loop by associating the cue and routine with a reward.

Habitual Behavior:

Over time, the habit loop becomes increasingly efficient. The basal ganglia take over more of the process, and the habit becomes a nearly automatic response to the cue. This is why habits can be so difficult to break, as they become deeply ingrained in our neural pathways.

Understanding the brain's role in habit formation provides insights into why habits can be challenging to change and how, with deliberate effort, we can rewire our brains to replace old habits with new, healthier ones. By working with the brain's natural processes, we can harness its incredible plasticity to create lasting change in our lives.

CHAPTER 10

How Small Changes Can Trigger Big Transformation

Small changes can trigger big transformations through the profound principle known as the domino effect. The essence of this concept lies in understanding how seemingly minor actions when consistently practiced, can set off a remarkable chain reaction of change. Here's how small changes can lead to significant transformations:

How easy it is to underestimate the importance of making little development consistently, and overestimate one defining moment. Frequently, we think within ourselves that great success requires great action. Whether it's writing a book, building a business, losing weight, or achieving any other goal, we always put pressure on ourselves

It is so easy to overestimate the importance of one defining moment and underestimate the value of making small improvements on a daily basis. Too often, we convince ourselves that massive success requires massive action. Whether it is losing weight, building a business, writing a book, winning a championship, or achieving any other goal, we put pressure on ourselves to make some earth-shattering improvement that everyone will talk about. Meanwhile, improving by 1 percent isn't particularly notable— sometimes it isn't even noticeable—but it can be far more meaningful, especially in the long run. The difference a tiny improvement can make over time is astounding. Here's how the math works out: if you can get 1 percent better each day for one year, you'll end up thirty-seven times better by the time you're done. Conversely, if you get 1 percent worse each day for one year, you'll decline nearly down to zero. What starts as a small win or a minor setback accumulates into something much more.

1% BETTER EVERY DAY 1% worse every day for one year. 0.99365 = 00.03 1% better every day for one year. 1.01365 = 37.78

The effects of small habits compound over time. For example, if you can get just 1 percent better each day, you'll end up with results that are nearly 37 times better after one year.

Habits are the compound interest of self-improvement. In the same way that money multiplies through compound interest, the effects of your habits multiply as you repeat them. They seem to make little difference on any given day and yet the impact they deliver over the months and years can be enormous. It is only when looking back two, five, or perhaps ten years later that the value of good habits and the cost of bad ones becomes strikingly apparent. This can be a difficult concept to appreciate in daily life. We often dismiss small changes because they don't seem to matter very much in the moment. If you save a little money now, you're still not a millionaire. If you go to the gym three days in a row, you're still out of shape. If you study Mandarin for an hour tonight, you still haven't learned the language. We make a few changes, but the results never seem to come quickly and so we slide back into our previous routines.

Unfortunately, the slow pace of transformation also makes it easy to let a bad habit slide. If you eat an unhealthy meal today, the scale doesn't move much. If you work late tonight and ignore your family, they will forgive you. If you procrastinate and put your project off until tomorrow, there will usually be time to finish it later. A single decision is easy to dismiss. But when we repeat 1 percent errors, day after day, by replicating poor decisions, duplicating tiny mistakes, and rationalizing little excuses, our small choices compound into toxic results. It's the accumulation of many missteps—a 1 percent decline here and there —that eventually leads to a problem. The impact created by a change in your habits is similar to the effect of shifting the route of an airplane by just a few degrees. Imagine you are flying from Los Angeles to New York City. If a pilot leaving from LAX adjusts the heading just 3.5 degrees south, you will land in Washington, D.C., instead of New York. Such a small change is barely noticeable at takeoff—the nose of the airplane moves just a few feet—but when magnified across the entire United States, you end up hundreds of miles apart. Similarly, a slight change in your daily habits can guide your life to a very different destination. Making a choice that is 1 percent better or 1 percent worse seems insignificant at the moment, but throughout moments that make up a lifetime, these choices determine the difference between who you are and who you could be. Success is the product of daily habits—not once-in-a-lifetime transformations. That said, it doesn't matter how successful or unsuccessful you are right now. What matters is whether your habits are putting you on the path toward success. You should be far more concerned with your current trajectory than with your current results. If you're a millionaire but you spend more than you earn each month, then you're on a bad trajectory. If your spending habits don't change, it's not going to end well. Conversely, if you're broke, but you save a little bit every month, then you're on the path toward financial freedom—even if you're moving slower than you'd like. Your outcomes are a lagging measure of your habits. Your net worth is a lagging measure of your financial habits. Your weight is a lagging measure of your eating habits. Your knowledge is a lagging measure of your learning habits. Your clutter is a lagging measure of your cleaning habits. You get what you repeat.

If you want to predict where you'll end up in life, all you have to do is follow the curve of tiny gains or tiny losses, and see how your daily choices will compound ten or twenty years down the line. Are you spending less than you earn each month? Are you making it to the gym each week? Are you reading books and learning something new each day? Tiny battles like these are the ones that will define your future self. Time magnifies the margin between success and failure. It will multiply whatever you feed it. Good habits make time your ally. Bad habits make time your enemy. Habits are a double-edged sword. Bad habits can cut you down just as easily as good habits can build you up, which is why understanding the details is crucial. You need to know how habits work and how to design them to your liking, so you can avoid the dangerous half of the blade.

Chapter 11

Introduction to Behavioral Transformation

Understanding the Foundations of Behavioral Health

Behavioral health is a multifaceted area that includes many facets of mental health, emotional stability, and social functioning. To understand the fundamentals of behavioral health, it is necessary to investigate the essential elements that contribute to an individual's mental and emotional condition.

Psychological elements:

Cognitive processes, emotions, and personality are all psychological elements that influence behavioral health. Understanding how people see and interpret their surroundings is critical to managing behavioral health issues. Thought patterns, coping techniques, and resilience all play an important part in molding one's mental health.

Social Determinants:

Social effects have a substantial impact on behavioral health. Family relationships, cultural background, social situation, and community support all have an influence on a person's mental health. Recognizing and treating these social variables is critical for building comprehensive behavioral health interventions.

Biological Influences:

The biological underpinnings of behavioral health include complicated interactions between genetics, neurobiology, and physiological components of mental health. Behavioral health disorders can be exacerbated by genetic predispositions, brain chemistry, and hormone imbalances. A thorough understanding of these biological aspects assists in the development of successful therapies.

Environmental Influence:

Environmental variables such as living circumstances,trauma exposure, and access to services all have a substantial impact on behavioral health.It is critical to foster a secure and supportive atmosphere in order to promote excellent mental health outcomes. Environmental stresses must be addressed in order to prevent and manage behavioral health issues.

Developmental Perspectives:

Behavioral health is dynamic and changes throughout time. Understanding behavioral health requirements at various phases of development, from childhood to maturity and beyond, enables tailored interventions. Developmental views shed light on age-related difficulties and possibilities for enhancing mental health.

Comprehensive Treatment strategy:

The foundations of behavioral health stress a comprehensive treatment strategy. Integrating psychological, social, biological, and environmental aspects enables a thorough knowledge of a person's behavioral health.To address the multidimensional character of mental health, holistic therapies include psychotherapy, medication, lifestyle changes, and community support.

Advocacy and Stigma Reduction:

Addressing societal stigma and pushing for mental health awareness are important aspects of behavioral health foundations.Promoting open discourse, education, and community involvement help to reduce stigma associated with mental health disorders, resulting in a more supportive and understanding society.

To summarize, comprehending the basis of behavioral health necessitates a careful examination of psychological, social, biological, and environmental components.A comprehensive strategy, along with education and advocacy, is the foundation of effective initiatives for improving behavioral health outcomes for people and communities alike.

The Role of Tiny Habits in Behavior Modification

Behavior modification is a dynamic topic within behavioral health that investigates techniques for bringing about beneficial changes in people's habits and routines.The notion of "Tiny Habits" has earned substantial attention in recent years as an effective and accessible method to behavior management.This book digs into the critical impact Tiny Habits have in molding and modifying habits for enhanced mental health and well-being.

Understanding Minor Habits:

Tiny Habits, a term coined by Stanford behavior scientist Dr. BJ Fogg, refers to the notion of making small, gradual adjustments in behavior to produce greater, long-term alterations. Tiny Habits, as opposed to radical changes, focuses on introducing achievable changes that are more likely to become ingrained in daily life.These can be as easy as sipping a glass of water, going for a brief stroll, or performing deep breathing exercises.

2.The Influence of Micro-Actions:

Tiny Habits is based on the idea that continuous, tiny activities may lead to large changes over time. This technique is particularly useful in the field of behavioral health since it corresponds with the progressive nature of habit building and makes the process more manageable for persons seeking change. Whether addressing stress management, sleep habits, or emotional regulation, including Tiny Habits helps individuals to make healthy behavioral improvements without feeling overwhelmed.

Tiny Habits' efficacy is dependent on the insertion of a cue-action-reward loop. Identifying a trigger or cue for the desired action, completing the Tiny Habit, and connecting it with a positive reward strengthens the habit loop. Taking a brief mindful breathing pause (activity) when feeling anxious (cue) and enjoying a sensation of tranquility (reward) builds a powerful and reinforcing habit.

Tiny Habits' versatility and personalization is one of its strengths in habit change. Tiny Habits may be tailored to fit an individual's lifestyle, hobbies, and goals, increasing the probability of long-term success. This tailored approach generates a sense of autonomy and empowerment, which are critical components in achieving beneficial behavioral changes.

Integration with 3.Traditional Therapeutic Approaches:

Tiny Habits supplement established therapy techniques in behavioral health.Tiny Habits, whether used alone or in conjunction with counseling, psychotherapy, or other therapies, provides individuals with practical skills for adopting and maintaining beneficial changes in their everyday lives.Tiny Habits and therapy techniques work together to provide a more holistic and complete approach to behavioral wellness.

Tiny Habits emerges as an important and accessible tool for habit change in the field of behavioral health. Individuals can begin on a positive transformation path that adds to overall mental well-being by leveraging the power of tiny, persistent activities. Integrating Tiny Habits into everyday routines provides a realistic and sustainable method to fostering healthy behaviors and creating long-term transformation in numerous parts of life.

Little Propensities for Better Actual Wellbeing

Drink a glass of water first thing.

We frequently don't get sufficient water in our frameworks, and get so occupied over the course of the day that we don't ponder halting to recharge ourselves. Or then again we renew with pop or espresso or tea yet not water.

Trigger yourself by forgetting about a major glass on the counter or table. Or on the other hand do what I do, and get a major travel mug with a cover. Around evening time, I top it off with a great deal of ice and a touch of water, and in the first part of the day it's hanging tight for me: a decent, cool cup of water. Flush the poisons, launch your framework, wake yourself up.

Park quite a distance from the entryway.

Battle the impacts of a single way of life by getting more strides into your day at whatever point you can. As a matter of fact, straightforward things like a more drawn out walk around the vehicle to the entryway may be more compelling than an energetic work-out at checking the impacts of extended periods of time at a work area.

Eat crude organic product or vegetables with each supper.

Consider this: a green side plate of mixed greens, a cut of melon, a few berries, a couple of carrot sticks and cucumber cuts. Not only will you get more supplements in, you will likewise be getting in more fiber and possibly assisting your body with shedding pounds, hold energy, and reducing hunger.

Stand up and extend consistently, at the top of the hour.

Trigger yourself with a signal on your telephone or watch or PC. Sitting for expanded time-frames is an impractical notion for both your body and your cerebrum. You want a psychological and actual break, and it doesn't need to be nothing to joke about. Stop, when your on-the-hour blare sounds at you. Stand up where you are, reach over your head, take a full breath, contact your toes, roll your shoulders. A little stretching will do you much good.

Convey a little sack of nuts or meat jerky wherever you go.

Something protein-rich will help fight off hunger as well as holding you back from arriving at that covetous moment that you'll eat anything in sight, irrespective of what the carbohydrate content is. Getting somewhat more protein in your eating regimen can assist with supporting your digestion and fabricate your muscle, also.

Chapter 12

Your Spiritual Challenge

A lot of people say that they don't have time to think spiritual thoughts. In fact, many don't even know what spirituality is. It is a sense of wellbeing that comes from being inspired by something that allows you to see beyond the surface. When you see a bird soar into the sky, it may fill you with wonder. When you see a rainbow, you may be reminded that there is a greater power looking over people or when you see the redness of a sunset, you may find yourself lost for words. All of these things help to make you a stronger and happier person, but if you don't take time to embrace them, you will not develop your spirituality and it's every bit as important to you as other areas of your life.

Habits that can be linked to spirituality could be anything. Let's show you an example.

Get out of bed – You do that every day and you don't need to think much about it.

Now let's add a potentially spiritual habit; Open the drapes and notice the color of the sky.

New Habit

You feel more at one with yourself and with nature.

There are loads of habits that can help you to feel more spiritual. I have added a list below and you can choose when to incorporate them into your life. Remember, this isn't a marathon. You add one habit to an existing habit. That doesn't mean a life changing goal or anything that is hard work. All it means is changing the routine a little bit by adding a new habit.

Chapter 13

Potentially good habits to add spirituality to your life

Switch off thoughts and be mindful for a moment – That means giving yourself one moment of calm in the storm. Look at what's around you and enjoy it. You could incorporate this into your eating routine by taking your time to enjoy the flavors and textures of what you eat, giving your mind a little calm.

New Habit

Be Mindful

Time taken: Less than five minutes

Result: You are more aware and less likely to think negative thoughts.

If your life is overflowing with activity, chances are that you don't sit down for any length of time and let your mind catch up with life. Meditation is great for this and it doesn't have to take too much time. Instead of thinking about your day, you think only about the breaths that you take and close your eyes to the world for a while. You can meditate for as little as five minutes and this makes your mind see the world in a much more positive light with more energy than you have experienced before, especially if you make it a daily habit.

Habit

Meditation

Time Spent: 5 minutes

Result: Clearer thought processes and ability to see things in a clearer way.

Perhaps you drive home every night and drive past somewhere that is potentially awesome. Why not add a new habit – Drive home – stop off at the beach. By doing this, you are following your initiative and allowing the spiritual side of your personality to have a little room to emerge.

New Habit

Stopping at an inspirational place

Time Spent: 15 minutes

Result: All positive habits that allow you more contact with nature result in being inspired and feed spirituality.

Spirituality doesn't mean going to church. It can mean that to some people. Lighting a candle in a church takes seconds and is very spiritual if you do so with sincerity. Adding little habits into your life that don't cost you a lot of time can make all the difference to your spiritual approach. You will know whether they are beneficial because they will make you feel positive about life. If they don't, try another one until you find those habits that encourage your spirituality to shine. Spirituality is something you feel inside. Allow your imagination to soar and to find habits that help you to develop this part of your own nature.

CHAPTER 14

HOW CAN HABITS CHANGE MY LIFE?

Habits can do so much to change your life. When you practice regular good habits, you're sure to see your life improving almost instantly. You will be more successful, and you will have more time to enjoy your favorite hobbies and activities as well. You might even find that you have a new purpose in life when you get through the fog of bad habits.

On the other hand, bad habits can cause more trouble that they're worth, especially in the long run. They can make you feel stressed, and can even lead to problems like obsessive-compulsive disorder in some cases. In order to make the most out of your life, you need to remove bad habits and concentrate on the good ones.

Breaking bad habits can cut back on stress

When you get rid of bad habits, you're ready to live a more stress-free lifestyle. Having bad habits can make you feel overwhelmed, especially when they take control of your life. You might feel like you need to perform your bad habit rituals on a regular basis, and you might not be able to stop them if you only try halfheartedly. Many bad habits that involve some sort of harm or damage to your body add to your stress even more, as you find more and more reasons to worry about your health.

Cut back on your bad habits to reduce the amount of stress in your life. The more bad habits you break, the freer you will feel, and the better off your will be emotionally. You will have less to worry about overall, and you will have more to feel good about every time you put another bad habit behind you.

Breaking bad habits can help you feel happier

Much like reducing your stress levels, breaking bad habits can make you feel better overall as well. Having a lot of bad habits is emotionally exhausting. It wears you down, and it makes you think you will never be able to come through the other side to a life filled with only good habits. It is important to remember that you are always able to try again, no matter what might have happened in the past, and that you will be able to find happiness with fewer bad habits in your life.

Some bad habits are serious enough to lead you toward depression and anxiety. In these situations, you might be on the road toward obsessive-compulsive disorder, or you might have other mental health issues you need to think about. The sooner you are able to stop repeating these bad habits, the happier you will be in the long run. Remember that no bad habit is so great that you cannot get beyond it with a little effort and planning.

Breaking bad habits can give you more time for activities you enjoy

Do you spend a lot of time smoking? Do you stop in the middle of your favorite TV shows to get up and find a snack? Are you often out of time to spend with your family because you waste time procrastinating instead? Every bad habit takes time out of your life that you could spend doing something else you enjoy more. There is no reason you need to spend so much time on your bad habits, and when you learn to break them, you have a lot more free time to spend however you choose.

Take Brendan for example. Brendan is a smoker, and he has been for most of his life. Every time he goes out with his family or friends, he has to stop in the middle of whatever he's doing and go have a smoke. Sometimes, he even leaves movie theaters or dinner dates to step outside for a cigarette. If Brendan could break this bad habit, he'd be able to spend more of his time with the people he enjoys being with, instead of standing alone outside smoking.

Starting good habits can help you succeed in life

Did you know that good habits can help you get ahead in life? When you have good habits to back you up, you can get a lot done in the workplace and around the house as well. More free time means you'll have more energy and mental stamina to devote to the things you need to get accomplished, and with good habits, you'll learn how to be better prepared for just about anything life can throw at you.

Let's look at Brendan again for this example. Smoking is a bad habit, but if he could stop smoking and replace that with a good habit, he might really improve his work. One good habit is reading a little bit every day and trying to learn something new. If Brendan takes the time he used to spend on smoke breaks reading and learning instead, he'll have more knowledge to help him succeed at work.

Starting good habits can get you organized

Good habits are great for helping you stay organized, as long as you don't go over the top with them. There are tons of different good habits that can help you get your life in order, like cleaning frequently, keeping track of your budget, planning family events on a calendar, and more. Keeping lists is another good habit to get into, especially when you frequently forget things or run late to your appointments.

Don't let keeping lists and making plans take the place of a bad habit in your life, however! If you get too worried about sticking to your plans, you'll wind up making yourself upset instead of using this skill for good. It's easy to fall into the trap of thinking negatively about your lists and calendars, so don't overdo it. Spend just a couple of minutes a day getting organized so you don't let it overtake your life.

Starting good habits can help you find a cause or goal in life

Finally, good habits can lead to something even greater if you give them a chance to. Maybe you spend a lot of time reading and learning, and you eventually learn about a cause that piques your interest. You might go from that into volunteering for a local branch of some support group, and from there, you may even find a new calling in life. Who knows? Your good habits give you plenty of chances to do something great with your life.

Samantha found out about her true calling in much the same way. When she was trying to educate herself on local organizations, she found out about one that helps terminally ill children take their dream vacations. She started volunteering, and in a few years, she was offered a job by the same group. She never expected her life to take that kind of turn, but she's never looked back since.

CHAPTER 15

CHALLENGE YOURSELF

There is always room for growth and personal development. Becoming successful and reaching new goals means moving forward. That entails always havingthe willingness to learn.

Whether you're saying yes to bigger responsibilities at work, doing things that once scared you, or you're just taking on a new challenge/ learning a new skill, make one of your goals specific to push yourself beyond the limits that you may have imagined.

This doesn't mean doing more every day or working yourself into the ground. It simply means not staying comfortable and doing things that are now easy.

You should always challenge yourself, and even if you choose something that isn't directly related to being successful in work, you will find that challenging yourself with something outside of your comfort zone, in any aspect of your life, will make you a more successful person.

As a leader, it's your job to take the reins and inspire change. But you can't reach your full potential unless you challenge yourself. By setting higher expectations--and striving to meet or exceed them--your productivity-boosting mentality can become contagious to all those around you.

Fortunately, I've been able to surround myself with leaders who consistently challenge themselves and motivate me to do the same.

Being able to see their constant desires to improve inspired me to never stop finding ways to grow and educate others.

Becoming an effective leader isn't a one-time goal. As you continue to brave uncertainty and build confidence in your abilities, challenge yourself, both personally and professionally, with these simple steps:

1. Start writing. Writing sounds basic, but putting pen to paper isn't always easy. It takes time, which often comes at a premium. When you have a spare moment, try to write and share your expertise. Actively thinking about your experiences and opinions can serve as a self-coaching session. However, don't write on a huge variety of topics. Write more about less. This forces you to think deeper into a specific topic and challenge your beliefs in manifesting what

you desire.

To get the ideas flowing, ask yourself what's important to write about. What do you want to achieve? What are the different steps and components that you need to know?

2. Narrow your expertise. The people who stand out are those who have built a reputation as the best. Challenge yourself to be the most knowledgeable in your discipline, and people will start to naturally think of you when seeking industry advice or thoughtful commentary. But don't get caught up in the same dry topics or you'll drive people away. Apply your expertise as a cornerstone to talk about a variety of different topics.

3. Constantly crave feedback. Gauging your performance through the eyes of others is one of

the best challenges--and often the most uncomfortable. That's why people tend to shy away from it, especially when they don't deliver. Take feedback not as an opportunity to earn approval, but as a chance to turn a perceived weakness into improvements making it a strength.

4. Be honest with yourself. Write down five skills you think are vital to the success that you desire. Then, grade yourself on each realistically. As you assess your abilities, take into account not only your own expectations, but also the expectations others might place on you. Once you have an idea, determine how you can improve the skills that will ultimately make you live in the practicum and not the ideology of it.

5. Set lofty goals. Some people will tell you to only set obtainable goals. But these are rarely challenging. Instead, shoot for something above

obtainable. You'll be surprised what you're capable of doing with endless possibilities.

6. You must choose the road that has not yet been travelled. I find it interesting when people do exactly what others are trying to accomplish in the niche of where their dreams stem from. Following is no way to become the leader you want to become. You must look for unexplored areas in your choice of expertise to help differentiate yourself from everyone else. What would that be for you?

7. Never stop learning. Knowledge is power. However, learning is a superpower. Adopting a student mentality pushes you to become a master of your craft. Reading is a huge way to achieve this. When you read, you're able to attain new found information that will inspire you to follow through your goals. Furthermore, you are

able to educate others on what you have learned. Don't keep what you know all to yourself. You must share your knowledge and be able to network with others achieve even greater possibilities. As you raise the bar for yourself, others will inevitably follow suit to your practices. Trust me, it's so contagious! And over time, you begin to make change to yourself and others around you just simply by being yourself. It's all about keeping your mindset on a higher vibrational level through simple thoughts and adapting to new, positive habits.

Chapter 16

Creating Productive Habits

Choose habits that align with your goals

On the road to achieving our goals, adopting habits that align with these objectives is a transformative process. Each goal you set for yourself is like a destination on a journey, and habits are like the steps you take to get there. If your steps take you in another direction, you will never reach your desired destination. Therefore, it is essential to choose habits that not only bring you closer to your goals, but are also compatible with your lifestyle and values.

First, identify your goals clearly and specifically. Ask yourself: What do I really want to achieve? Your goals can be professional, such as career advancement, or personal, such as improving your health. Once you are clear about your goals, the next step is to establish habits that will help you achieve them. For example, if your goal is to improve your physical health, a relevant habit might be to exercise regularly.

The next step is to do an honest analysis of your current habits. Ask yourself: Are my daily activities moving me closer to my goals or further away from them? This self-assessment exercise will help you identify habits you need to modify or eliminate. For example, if you spend a lot of time on social media and your goal is to write a book, this habit may be diverting your attention and energy away from your main goal.

Once you have identified the habits you need to adopt, start integrating them into your daily routine gradually. Don't try to change everything overnight. For example, if you want to incorporate reading into your daily routine, start with a few minutes each day and increase the time gradually. The key is consistency. Habits get stronger with repetition

It's also important to surround yourself with an environment that supports your new habits. If your goal is to eat healthier, having a kitchen full of nutritious options will facilitate this habit. Likewise, if you surround yourself with people who share your goals and habits, it will be easier for you to maintain these behaviors.

Another useful strategy is to link your new habits to activities you already do regularly. For example, if you want to start meditating and you are already in the habit of having a cup of coffee every morning, try meditating right after your coffee. This method, known as "habit building," can be very effective in incorporating new routines into your life.

Finally, it is essential that you reward yourself for small accomplishments along the way to adopting new habits. Not only will this keep you motivated, but it will also reinforce the habit. Rewards can be as simple as taking a moment to acknowledge your progress or giving yourself a small treat after a week of sticking to your new habit.

In summary, choosing and maintaining habits that align with your goals is a dynamic process that requires self-awareness, planning and patience. Remember that every little habit adds up and brings you one step closer to your goals. With commitment and consistency, the habits you choose will be fundamental pillars in your journey to success and self-fulfillment.

Techniques for establishing new habits

To establish new habits, it is essential to first understand what they are and how they work. Habits are automatic behaviors or routines that we perform with little or no conscious thought. They are formed through repetition and, once ingrained, can significantly influence our daily behavior and overall productivity. Therefore, adopting productive habits can have a transformative impact on our lives.

The first step in establishing a new habit is to identify a clear and concrete goal. This goal should be specific, measurable, attainable, relevant and time-bound (SMART). For example, instead of saying "I want to be fit," a SMART goal might be "I want to exercise for 30 minutes a day, five days a week." Having a clear, well-defined goal helps focus your efforts and gives you a clear yardstick to measure your progress.

Once you have a clear goal, the next step is to break it down into small, manageable actions. This approach makes it easier to manage change, as large goals can be overwhelming. For example, if your goal is to exercise regularly, you might start by walking 10 minutes a day and gradually increase the duration or intensity of your physical activity.

Creating a favorable environment is another important aspect of establishing new habits. The environment plays a crucial role in habit formation, as it can act as a trigger for both positive and negative behaviors. For example, if you want to develop the habit of reading more, you could place a book in a visible place where you usually relax. In this way, the book becomes a visual and accessible reminder of your new habit.

Positive reinforcement is another key technique. It involves rewarding yourself in some way after performing the desired activity. This reward does not have to be large or expensive; it can be something as simple as taking a few minutes to relax or enjoying a small treat. Positive reinforcement helps associate the new habit with a pleasant experience, increasing the likelihood that you will repeat it in the future.

Consistency is also crucial for habit formation. Performing the activity regularly, preferably at the same time each day, helps to cement the habit. For example, if you decide to exercise in the morning, try to do it at the same time every day. This helps your brain associate that specific time with the activity of exercising.

In addition, it is important to be patient and compassionate with yourself. Habit formation is a process that takes time and it's normal to have days when you don't meet your set goals. Instead of being hard on yourself or discouraged, recognize that forming a new habit is a challenge and celebrate the small accomplishments along the way.

Finally, keeping a record of your progress can be very useful. Writing down your successes and difficulties allows you to see how you are evolving over time and provides you with valuable information to make adjustments if necessary. It can also be a source of motivation to continue, as it allows you to see the progress you have made.

Forming new habits requires a combination of clear and specific goals, small and manageable actions, a supportive environment, positive reinforcement, consistency, patience and self-compassion, and progress monitoring. By applying these techniques, you can develop productive habits that will help you achieve your goals and improve your quality of life.

Maintaining consistency

On the road to adopting productive habits, one of the biggest challenges is maintaining consistency. Often, we start out with enthusiasm, but over time, that initial momentum can wane. To prevent this from happening, we need to develop strategies that help us stay focused and committed to our long-term goals.

First, it is important to remember why we choose to adopt these habits. Each habit we incorporate should have a clear purpose and be aligned with our personal and professional goals. By keeping the 'why' behind each habit in mind, we can reignite our motivation when it begins to wane.

An effective technique for maintaining consistency is to set reminders and alerts. These act as cues that remind us to perform our usual routines. These alerts can be as simple as a sticky note on the mirror or an alarm on the phone. The important thing is that they serve as a constant reminder of our intentions.

In addition, consistency is strengthened by creating an enabling environment. This involves organizing our physical and digital space in a way that supports our habits. For example, if one of our habits is to read more, having a book always at hand in our resting place can be of great help. Similarly, if we want to reduce the time we spend on social networks, we could consider removing these applications from the main screen of our phone.

Tracking our progress is another fundamental pillar of maintaining consistency. Keeping a record of our habits allows us to see our progress and celebrate small achievements, which is a great motivator. We can use anything from a simple planner to specialized apps to keep track. Seeing how we have been able to maintain a habit over time can give us an extra boost to keep going.

Flexibility also plays an important role in maintaining consistency. Sometimes, rigidity in our plans can lead to failure. We must be willing to adjust our habits according to our life circumstances. For example, if we have committed to exercise every morning but a change in our work schedule makes it impractical, we might consider shifting our exercise sessions to the afternoon.

In addition, it is crucial to learn to deal with deviations without being too hard on ourselves. We all have days when we deviate from our habits. Instead of criticizing ourselves, it is important to analyze what caused the deviation and how we can avoid it in the future. This compassionate and reflective attitude will help us get back on track without becoming demotivated.

Associating with people who share similar goals can go a long way toward keeping us on track. Whether it's a gym buddy, a book club, or an online group, having a supportive community can increase our chances of success. Not only do these people offer us motivation and advice, but they can also be a source of accountability.

Finally, it is important to remember that habit adoption is a constantly evolving process. What works today may not be effective tomorrow, so we must be open to experimentation and change. As we grow and change, our habits must also evolve to reflect who we are and where we want to go.

Maintaining consistency in our habits requires a balance between self-discipline and self-compassion. We need to set reminders, create enabling environments, track our progress, be flexible, learn from deviations, seek support from others and be open to change. By implementing these strategies, we will not only be able to maintain our habits, but also enjoy the process and see results in our lives.

Chapter 17

Identifying Bad Habits

Recognizing Barriers to Change

Before we start building good habits, it's important to identify and understand the bad habits that may be keeping us from reaching our full potential. This chapter is dedicated to exploring bad habits, how to recognize them, and why they are so challenging to break.

What Are Bad Habits?

Bad habits are unwanted behaviors that repeatedly harm our health, happiness, or productivity. They can range from unhealthy habits like smoking or overeating to unproductive behaviors like procrastination or wasting time on social media. Identifying these habits is the first step towards positive change.

Recognizing Bad Habits

1. Self-awareness: The first step to recognizing bad habits is self-awareness. Stop and reflect on your daily behaviors. What actions do you automatically take, even if you know they are harmful? For example, maybe you smoke or bite your nails when you're stressed.

2. Feedback from Others: Sometimes our friends, family or colleagues can recognize our bad habits before we do. Be open to constructive feedback and ask those close to you about behaviors they find problematic.

3. Negative Consequences: Observe the negative consequences of your habits. Bad habits often result in physical, emotional or social problems. For example, excessive alcohol consumption can lead to health problems and damaged relationships.

Why are Bad Habits Hard to Break?

Understanding why bad habits are persistent is key to overcoming them. Some reasons why they are difficult to let go of include:

- Immediate Rewards: Many bad habits offer immediate rewards, even if they are harmful in the long term. For example, eating sweets can provide instant pleasure but lead to health problems.

- Ingrained Habits: The longer we practice a bad habit, the more ingrained it becomes in our daily routine.

- Compensatory Effect: Sometimes we resort to bad habits to deal with stress or negative emotions, creating a vicious cycle.

- Lack of Alternatives: If we don't have healthy alternatives or coping strategies, we are more likely to continue with bad habits.

Conclusion

Identifying bad habits is the first step to positive change. Be aware of your behaviors and how they affect your life. Remember that changing habits is a gradual process. In the next chapter, we'll explore how to set effective goals for forming new habits and how to replace bad habits with healthier, more productive behaviors.

You are on the right path to significant personal transformation. We will continue to discover how small changes can lead to big results in your life.

What are the main components of a habit?

This is necessary so that we clearly understand how, from which bricks we can develop the very habit that we want to form, how to make it quickly entrenched in our life.

Our habits are a kind of reaction of our psyche to a certain action. Thus, it is necessary to create a certain situation, when a certain action is accomplished, connected with this situation and the surrounding conditions.

An individual with a certain habit seems to be focused on the corresponding action and will certainly perform this action as soon as the opportunity presents itself.

Any habits, both bad and good, consist of three components: trigger, action and reward.

Trigger

A trigger, also called a signal or stimulus, is what causes our habit.

For example, take the habit of banging your nails on the table. The trigger in this will often be a stressful situation, the action - actually banging the nails, and the reward - a sense of calm and ability to concentrate.

The trigger is most often some kind of previous action, setting, time, or emotion.

Action - for example, in the morning we get up and go to have a shower, the telephone will ring and we will respond.

The trigger "action" is a very useful thing for the formation of new habits. We can create a whole set of habits, developing them one by one and consistently connecting them with each other.

Many habits are tied to the place. We come to such a place and always do the same thing.

For example, we come to work and sit down at the computer, come home and go to the kitchen to drink tea with cookies, or the husband comes home from work and lies down on the sofa in front of the TV. Thus, the place and the environment influences what behavior follows after we get there.

Time is one of the most frequent triggers. We all know, for example, evening habits: when in the evening we go to brush our teeth, put the phone on charge and lie down.

Emotions are very strong triggers and the most dangerous. Such emotional states as depression, boredom, resentment, anger often cause our negative habits.

The boss shouted at you? You urgently need to smoke a cigarette. It doesn't matter that you don't smoke for a week.

Have a falling out with your loved one? You urgently need to eat something tasty like a piece of cake and better two. It doesn't matter that you on the diet for losing weight.

In addition, triggers can be completely different things.

For example, you saw something, and it worked right away.

You saw a notification from the contact - immediately there was a desire to open it, to respond (word after word and imperceptibly flew a couple of hours).

You saw a red light at a traffic light before crossing the road - right there you stopped by the habit; you didn't even have time to think about stopping on the red light. You just took out of pocket the phone and stopped without a second thought. Or you felt some kind of smell, heard something - it can also cause familiar reactions in you.

Whether we admit it or not, we have a million habits and they are tied to a million triggers. Some of these triggers are very strong and perform the same actions; others are not so strong and can only incline us to one or another action. Both triggers can be reprogrammed to create a strong link between them and the habits that we need.

Action

As you have noticed, a trigger causes a reaction or action.

The action may be physical, mental or emotional.

The above examples, I hope, have already convinced you that after some kind of trigger works, there is always some action.

Reward

And the last essential component of habit is reward.

Reward allows the brain to remember one or another habit for the future.

For example, a man came to the store for juice. His favorite juice was not, and he bought another.

The wife was very happy and grateful, as it turned out to be her favorite juice. The next time the same thing happened. Habit formation began. Bought juice - received praise.

Instead of a wife there can be a supervisor, instead of juice, overtime, instead of praise, a bonus.

After the action of any habit, whether it is positive or negative, there is always a reward. Even if this habit is absolutely harmful, there is always some kind of reward that reinforces this habit.

There is never a habit without a reward. It happens that this reward is not obvious, it can be in the form of a moment of peace or a slight feeling of satisfaction that we have after the action.

Thus, any habit consists of a trigger or stimulus, action and reward, regardless of whether it is a good habit or a bad one.

I recommend that you read it again or even write it down somewhere, because it is really very important. Further, when you will create your habits, you will practice and reinforce them - all this will be based on these three components.

In the next chapter, you will learn on what conditions you will be able to perform a specific action or not. This will help you to review your past actions when you tried to introduce some habit into your life, but you didn't succeed. And you will understand why this did not work. Perhaps at this stage you will have thoughts on how to fix it, and if not, after reading all the chapters, they will definitely appear.

Chapter 18

The Power of Rituals and Keystone Habits

In this chapter, we will explore the power of rituals and keystone habits in shaping our routines and fostering personal transformation. By understanding how to create purposeful rituals and identify impactful keystone habits, we can unlock the potential for positive cascades of change in various areas of our lives.

Morning and Evening Rituals

Establishing morning and evening rituals can set the tone for our day and promote overall well-being. These rituals serve as anchors to our day, providing structure and intentionality to our routines.

Creating purposeful morning rituals involves:

- Setting Intentions: Starting the day by reflecting on our goals and affirming our intentions for the day ahead. This can be done through journaling, visualization, or affirmation exercises.

- Energizing Activities: Incorporating activities that energize and invigorate us, such as exercise, meditation, or reading uplifting materials. Engaging in these activities early in the day can boost mood and productivity.

- Prioritizing Self-Care: Allocating time for self-care activities that nourish our physical, mental, and emotional well-being. This can include activities like taking a relaxing bath, practicing mindfulness, or enjoying a nutritious breakfast.

Creating purposeful evening rituals involves:

- Reflection and Gratitude: Reflecting on the events of the day and expressing gratitude for the positive experiences. This can be done through journaling or simply taking a few moments to mentally acknowledge blessings and achievements.

- Wind-Down Activities: Engaging in relaxing activities to signal to our bodies and minds that it's time to unwind and prepare for restful sleep. This can include reading a book, practicing gentle stretching, or practicing a calming mindfulness exercise.

- Quality Sleep Environment: Creating a serene sleep environment by minimizing distractions and ensuring optimal comfort. This can involve keeping electronic devices out of the bedroom, adjusting lighting and temperature, and using comfortable bedding.

By incorporating purposeful morning and evening rituals into our lives, we cultivate a sense of balance, intention, and well-being that can positively affect our entire day.

Keystone Habits: Unleashing Domino Effects

Keystone habits are powerful behaviors that have the potential to unleash a cascade of positive changes across different areas of our lives. These habits act as the foundation for other habits and can have a profound impact on our overall well-being.

Identifying keystone habits involves:

- Self-Reflection: Reflecting on our current habits and identifying behaviors that have a notable influence on other areas of our lives. These habits may serve as catalysts for change and contribute to our desired personal transformation.

- Examining Habits' Ripple Effects: Observing how a particular habit affects other aspects of our lives. For example, regular exercise may not only improve physical health but also enhance mental well-being, leading to increased productivity and better relationships.

- Experimentation and Adaptation: Trying out new habits that have the potential to be keystone habits and evaluating their effects over time. It's essential to embrace a growth mindset and adapt our habits as we learn what works best for us.

By identifying and nurturing keystone habits, we can experience transformative changes that extend far beyond the specific habit itself. These habits act as catalysts, setting off a series of positive domino effects that amplify our personal growth and well-being.

In the upcoming chapters, we will delve further into overcoming obstacles, building resilience, and creating sustainable habits. By understanding and implementing these strategies, we can strengthen our habits and continue on the path of lasting personal transformation. So, let's continue this journey with excitement and embrace the power of rituals and keystone habits!

Chapter 19

Neurology, Willpower and Habit Change

Percentages differ. Some claim that, on average, only 88% of New Year's resolutions made each year fail. Others say the failure rate is around 92%. But whether it is 88% or 92%, the failure rate is still rather alarming. This prompts us to ask why only 8-10% of millions of people who desire to change their lives succeed in the endeavor. What separates the 8-10% successful people from the rest?

Because of these intriguing figures, psychologists from different parts of the world have conducted studies to understand the phenomenon. These studies gave way to scientific explanations on why people fail when they resolve to change multiple habits at a time. Neurology has also provided suggestions on how a person can change his life for the better.

Why the Human Brain Cannot Handle Multiple Habit Changes

There is no doubt that willpower is the key to successful life changes. We often here people refer to successful people as strong-willed, committed or determined. What makes a person strong-willed or weak-willed?

The part of the brain that controls willpower is located in the prefrontal cortex – the area right behind the forehead. The brain cells in the prefrontal cortex are pretty busy in our daily lives because on top of controlling willpower, they also control our short-term memory, how we solve abstract problems and how we stay focused. You can just imagine how the prefrontal cortex juggles several tasks at a time.

Scientific studies have shown that when the prefrontal cortex is pretty occupied, our willpower is correspondingly diminished. This concept is better explained by the experiment performed by Prof. Baba Shiv:

"A group of undergraduate students were divided into 2 groups. One group was given a two-digit number to remember. The other was given a seven-digit number to remember. Then, after a short walk through the hall, they were offered the choice between two snacks: a slice of chocolate cake or a bowl of fruit. What's most surprising: The students with 7-digit numbers to remember were twice as likely to pick the slice of chocolate compared to the students with the 2-digits. Those extra numbers took up valuable space in the brain – they were a "cognitive load" – making it much harder to resist a decadent dessert."

Though this scientific explanation is quite revealing, it has not diminished the fact that human beings can still achieve greatness and success in life.

Instead, it has pointed us toward another revelation that like any muscle in the human body, we can train the prefrontal cortex to better control our willpower.

Based on Prof. Baba Shiv's experiment, we cannot force our prefrontal cortex to handle multiple habit changes at a time. This is like asking your body to run a complete marathon when you have never jogged or run in your life.

Here is a simple training plan to improve the performance of your prefrontal cortex:

Start with only one habit change.

Pushing your brain beyond its limit or "cognitive overload", as Prof. Shiv calls it, only leads to failure and frustrations. To prevent this, decide to change only one habit so you can focus all your energies to accomplish this.

Take baby steps.

After you've chosen the habit you want to change, you need to analyze it further to break it down to smaller, bite-size pieces. Stating your goal in general terms is just like having several goals at a time. Your prefrontal cortex will need to process a broad concept that could lead to "cognitive overload".

To increase your likelihood of success, assign the simplest task to your prefrontal cortex. Instead of saying you want to lose weight, you can say "I will go for a 10 minute jog every evening after work." This new habit may seem irrelevant but once

www.ingramcontent.com/pod-product-compliance
Lightning Source LLC
LaVergne TN
LVHW021239080526
838199LV00088B/4733